DR.

EASY WAY TO

STOP

SMOKING

Shobi Nolan

Copyright © 2020 By Shobi Nolan

No part of this book may be reproduced in any form, or by any electronic or mechanical means without prior permission from the author, except in the case of brief quotations in articles and reviews.

Contents

CHAPTER 1	1
INTRODUCTION	1
Central Nervous System	4
Respiratory System	5
Cardiovascular System	7
Integumentary System	8
Digestive System	8
Reproductive System	9
CHAPTER 2	10
DR. SEBI DIET	10
Dr. Sebi Alkaline Diet	14
The Dr. Sebi Diet Guide	16
CHAPTER 3	19
HOW SMOKING DESTROYS THE BODY	19
Circulation	20
Heart	21

Stomach	23
Skin	23
Bones	24
Brain	24
Lungs	26
Mouth And Throat	27
Reproduction And Fertility	28
CHAPTER 4	30
HOW TO QUIT SMOKING	30
Why Quitting Is Hard	30
Your Quit Plan Matters A Lot	33
Things You Need To Do Before You Start In Order To Set Yourself Up For Success	36
Dr. Sebi Diet Guide To Manage Common Triggers	44
How To Manage Cravings	49

Dr. Sebi Guide To Manage Nicotine Withdrawal Symptoms 51

CHAPTER 5 — 54
MUCUS CLEANSE — 54

What Is Mucus? — 54

Mucus And Body Health — 56

Causes Of Mucus Buildup In The Body: — 58

Easy Guide For Mucus Cleanse — 61

CHAPTER 6 — 67
DR. SEBI APPROVED HERBS AND VEGETABLES — 67

CHAPTER 7 — 192
DR SEBI FOOD LIST — 192

Vegetables — 193

Fruits — 194

Spices and Seasonings — 195

Grains — 196

Sugars and Sweeteners	196
Herbal Teas	196
Nuts and Seeds	197
Oils	197

CHAPTER 1

INTRODUCTION

Using pipe, cigar, or maybe hookah as substitutes for cigarettes doesn't save one from all the associated health risks. Most of the ingredients used to make cigarettes are found in hookahs and cigars. Thus, they are not safe routes.

According to the American Lungs Association, about 600 ingredients are used to produce cigarettes and these substances generate over 7,000 chemicals when they burn. Among the toxic chemicals produced, over 69 are linked to cancer.

Research by the Centers for Disease Control and Prevention (CDC) shows that smoking is one of the most common preventable cause of death. The United States has recorded the mortality rate of smokers to be three times that of nonsmokers.

Though most of the health complications associated with smoking are not immediate, the effects can last until death, if not stopped earlier. So, the best way to avoid these problems is by quitting.

There is no way to smoke cigarettes that is not dangerous to your health. No single substance in the tobacco products is safe for you. All the substances in tobacco, including nicotine, acetone, tar, carbon monoxide (CO), etc. are dangerous to your health. They go far beyond the lungs to affect the whole body.

There are varieties of complications associated with smoking. Though most of these effects are long-term, there are some health effects that are immediate. It is pertinent to learn some of these symptoms and health complications that one may encounter as a result of smoking.

Central Nervous System

Nicotine is one of the major ingredients used to produce cigarettes. As a mood-altering drug, it gets to your brain in seconds and makes you feel energized.

Unfortunately, this feeling doesn't last for long, which makes smokers crave for more when they start feeling tired again - leading to addiction and difficult to quit.

Attempt to withdraw from nicotine can make one feel irritated, anxious, and depressed, with impaired cognitive function. It can also cause headaches and make it difficult for one to sleep. But, all these are temporary and will wean away with time.

Respiratory System

Smoking can damage the lungs in many ways. Even inhaling smoke puts one at risk. Some of the chronic irreversible damage that smoking can cause are:

- Chronic bronchitis - permanent inflammation of the lungs breathing tube lining.

- Emphysema - damage to the air sac of the lungs.

- Chronic obstructive pulmonary disease(COPD) - varieties of lung diseases.

- Lung cancer

- Asthma etc.

As one gets addicted and impacts the functioning of the lungs, attempting to withdraw may cause respiratory discomfort and congestion. The airways and lungs begin to heal which most times increases the production of mucus.

Cardiovascular System

The nicotine in cigarettes restricts blood flow by making the blood vessels tighten. This can damage the whole cardiovascular system. Continuous narrowing of the blood vessels for a long time can lead to peripheral artery disease.

Moreover, smoking increases blood pressure, and blood clots. It as well weakens the walls of the blood vessel. These effects together can increase the risk of stroke. The risk is higher if you have had heart attack before, or heart bypass surgery.

Integumentary System

Smoking affects the skin in so many ways. A research revealed that smoking increases the risk of skin cancer (squamous cell carcinoma). Moreover, your nails are exposed to fungal infections.

Digestive System

Larynx, esophagus, throat, mouth, and pancreatic cancer are among the health risks of smoking. Smoking also increases the risk of type 2 diabetes as it affects the insulin.

Reproductive System

The nicotine in cigarettes can lower the rate of blood flow into the genital area. This can lead to low sexual performance in men and decreased lubrication and satisfaction in women.

CHAPTER 2

DR. SEBI DIET

Dr. Sebi's alkaline diet is a plant-based diet that helps to eliminate toxic wastes from the body and rejuvenate body cells.

The alkaline diet relies strictly on a list of plant foods and products approved by Dr. Sebi. Through his diet, Dr. Sebi did great wonders in people's lives; cured many diseases and revived complicated health conditions. In fact, it is one of the best plant-based diets. It was listed as one of the most popular diets in 2019.

If we can eat delicious meals and free our body from diseases, what again are we looking for? Dr. Sebi's diet can help you detox your body completely, including mucus removal, liver cleansing, diabetes reversal, cancer treatment, lupus and herpes cure, etc. Learn how to eat good foods, and you may not need medications to stay healthy.

You don't need medications to cleanse mucus from your body when you can easily get rid of it naturally by drinking and eating the right foods. By so doing, you can simply prevent and/or manage high blood pressure. The foods to take good care of your condition can be found in the nearest local grocery store.

Prepare your mind and stock your kitchen with the right foods from Dr. Sebi Approved List. Then follow the instructions in the book to help you quit smoking.

But before we get started, let's look at Dr. Sebi and his diet.

Who is Dr. Sebi?

Alfredo Darlington Bowman is an African herbalist who developed an alkaline plant diet that is based on bio-mineral balance theory. Though he is not a certified medical doctor or a Ph.D. holder, he is widely known as Dr. Sebi.

His diet is named after his popular name, The Dr. Sebi Diet. His diet was developed for those that wish to naturally detox their body for total wellness and prevent diseases by eating approved healthy plant foods.

Dr. Sebi claimed that our body is protected from diseases when it is in an alkaline state. According to him, acidic state of the body and mucus buildup in the body are the major causes of various diseases.

Though there is no scientific backup, Dr. Sebi claimed that his diet has the potential to cure lupus, sickle cell anemia, AIDS, and leukemia. He believes his diet could completely restore alkalinity in the body and detoxify the whole body.

Dr. Sebi Alkaline Diet

Dr. Sebi's diet is regarded as a vegan diet since it is a completely plant-based diet. No animal product is allowed in the diet.

Dr. Sebi claimed that this diet can make the body heal itself completely from diseases. Though there is no scientific proof for this, a lot of people who are on the diet have attested to the claim.

As a result, Dr. Sebi's diet is ranked one of the most popular diets in 2019.

The Dr. Sebi Diet Guide

Dr. Sebi's diet is solely based on plants and supplements approved by Dr. Sebi.

The diet guide can be found on his website. The simple rules to follow on Dr. Sebi diet are;

- Only foods and products listed in the nutritional guide are to be consumed.

- You must drink at least 1 gallon of water every day (that is about 3.8 liters).

- If you are on any medication, you have to take your Dr. Sebi supplements, at least, one hour before your medication.

- You don't take alcohol.
- You must not eat any animal products.
- Don't use the microwave to prepare your foods.
- Only consume naturally grown grains as listed in the guide. No wheat product is allowed.
- No seedless fruit and no canned food is permitted.

Moreover, you are expected to be using Dr. Sebi's supplements to support your diet.

CHAPTER 3

HOW SMOKING DESTROYS THE BODY

A report from research has shown that one in every two smokers end up dying from diseases that are related to smoking. Cancers start from mutations. And for each 15 sticks of cigarettes you smoke, you cause mutation to your body.

If only smokers could see the damage they are causing to their own body, they would not need any advice or motivation to quit smoking.

Circulation

The tar in cigarettes contain poisonous chemicals. Smoking facilitates the entering of these chemicals in the blood.

- Smoking makes the blood to become thick and that increases clot formation.

- Smoking makes the heart overwork itself by increasing heart rate and blood pressure.

- Smoking lowers the amount of oxygen rich blood in circulation by narrowing the arteries.

All these changes together can cause stroke and heart attack.

Heart

Smoking increases the risk of coronary heart disease, stroke, cerebrovascular disease, peripheral vascular disease, and heart attack. Once blood circulation is reduced and the heart damaged, the person is exposed to various heart diseases.

The nicotine and carbon monoxide from cigarettes make the heart work faster and that alone puts strain on it. Other components of cigarette smoke cause damage to the lining of the coronary artery.

Research revealed that smoking doubles the risk of heart attack, and smokers have doubled risk of dying from coronary heart disease than non-smokers.

However, smokers can still escape all these health risks by quitting smoking. Quitting reduces the risks to half after one year. Interestingly, after 15 years of not smoking, the risk will be the same with someone that never smoked.

Stomach

Smoking can lead to acid reflux. Smoking weakens the muscles of the lower end of the oesophagus, and thus, causing acid to flow back up into the oesophagus. Moreover, smoking can as well cause ulcers and stomach cancer.

Research has shown that taking 10 - 20 cigarettes or more a day increases the risk of kidney cancer by 2.

Skin

Since smoking lowers oxygen flow to the skin, it makes the skin to look grey, dull, and age faster than normal. The toxins in the body as a result of smoking cause cellulite.

Bones

Smoking can lead to osteoporosis, where the bones appear to be weak and brittle. This is more prevalent in women.

Brain

Smokers have higher risk of dying from stroke because smoking increases the risk of stroke by 50%. Stroke is one of the health challenges that damage the brain and consequently lead to death.

As the walls of the blood vessels become weak as a result of smoking, it starts to build up bulge in the blood vessel. This bulge is what causes brain aneurysm. Once the bulge bursts or ruptures, it can cause extreme health conditions, a type of stroke widely known as subarachnoid haemorrhage. This stroke damages the brain and leads to death.

Research has shown that by stopping smoking one can reduce the high risk to half after one year. Then after staying for 5 years without smoking, the risk is completely lowered to the same level with someone that has never smoked.

Lungs

Smoking can affect the lungs badly. Beyond colds, coughs, asthma, smoking can lead to fatal health conditions like emphysema, pneumonia, and lung cancer. Smoking causes 83% and 84% of deaths from chronic obstructive pulmonary disease (COPD) and lung cancer respectively.

Chronic obstructive pulmonary disease (COPD) is a collection of progressive and debilitating lung diseases. Symptoms of COPD include difficult breathing, cough and frequent chest infection.

Mouth And Throat

Smoking can cause oral thrush. Moreover, issues like stained teeth, bad breath, gum disease, and damage to taste bud are associated with smoking. The most dreadful implications of smoking is the cancer associated with it, which could be cancer in the tongue, voice box, esophagus, lips, and throat. In fact, smoking is the root cause of 93% of all recorded oropharyngeal cancers.

Quitting smoking and staying for 20 years without smoking will reduce all these risks to the level the same with someone who has never smoked.

Reproduction And Fertility

Research has shown that smoking can reduce sperm count, damage sperm, and lead to testicular cancer. Men who smoke have very low sperm count compared to those that do not smoke.

Smoking can cause cervical cancer and infertility in women. Smoking makes it difficult to get rid of human papillomavirus infection from the body. This can result in cancer. For pregnant women, smoking can cause miscarriage and stillbirth.

CHAPTER 4

HOW TO QUIT SMOKING

Why Quitting Is Hard

It is easier said than done. It is not easy to break a habit, especially when the body and mind has been configured to fit into a particular pattern of life. Though we know the health implications associated with smoking, it's still not easy to break the habit. Many have tried and failed. At the same time, many have succeeded in kicking the habit. The only truth here is that quitting smoking is really difficult to do.

Smoking cigarettes leads to both a psychological and a physical addition. The nicotine in cigarettes is highly addictive as it usually gives the smoker an instant "feel good" effect. Many people go for cigarette anytime they feel stressed, depressed, weak, bored, etc. Attempting to stop it when one is already addicted causes withdrawal symptoms and cravings.

To some, smoking has turned to a daily ritual. A right they need to perform at a specific time of the day. Some are addicted to taking it after every meal. Some take it with coffee. Some go for it during their break time. Some also take it for different reasons.

No matter how, where, when, and why someone smokes, there is a good personal reason that prompted that action in the first place. No one just smokes cigarettes to die from it. We all have good personal reasons why we do things.

Going back to the root cause of our actions goes a long way in helping us solve the problem. If we can remember why we started smoking or why we still smoke today, we can quick the habit by searching for an alternative means that is effective, and healthy to our body.

To succeed in quitting smoking, the person needs to address all issues including the reason that promoted you to smoke, the feeling, cravings, routine, addiction, etc. Knowing all these and strategizing a suitable quit plan can help one to break the habit easily.

Your Quit Plan Matters A Lot

Some people have successfully quit smoking by going cold turkey right from day one. Also, many have stopped smoking by using plans and guides. Whichever way that works for you is fine as long as the plan is healthy and safe for you.

Trying to do something at a given time may not actually be difficult as doing the same thing for a long period of time. Quitting smoking can be done but how long can you handle the challenges that go with it? Some have tried it for days and weeks and ended up going back to where they started from.

However, coping with the short term challenges is not more important than the long term challenges. So, the best strategy to stop smoking is to think long term. Can you do it for a week, a month, or three? Long-term plan is the bedrock of complete withdrawal. But it doesn't end there. There are important questions you need to ask to help you handle some challenge that might arise along the line.

Here are some questions to ponder on before you start.

- Am I a heavy smoker or just a social smoker? Is one nicotine patch enough for me?

- Knowing the type of smoker you are will go a long way in helping you organize the best plan.

- Are there certain events, activities, people, or places I can associate with my smoking habit?

- Do I always have the urge to smoke before and/or after any meal. Do I smoke each time I take a drink?

- What are those feelings that make me crave for cigarettes?

Things You Need To Do Before You Start In Order To Set Yourself Up For Success

Tell people around you what you are up to.

Let those around you know what your plan is and it will help you a lot in the journey. You need support and care because it's not always an easy journey, especially when you are doing it alone.

So, tell your family, friends, and colleagues what you are up to and how they can help you to achieve maximum success. You can also find someone that wants to stop smoking and with the person. At least, you will encourage each other.

Set a suitable date to quit

You need to prepare your mind before you start the journey. So choose a date you think will work best for you.

Prepare for the challenge

Definitely, temptations will come along the line. You will see yourself in situations that will force you to give up. If you did not prepare your mind before starting, you may end up giving up. Then think of the cravings and withdrawal effects that you will encounter along the process. Prepare and plan how to overcome those challenges. Thanks to the Dr. Sebi diet. We will discuss this and how to handle these challenges using the Dr. Sebi diet and products.

Declutter

Clean up your living spaces and office place. Remove everything that has connection with cigarettes such as lighters, cigarettes, cigarette packs, ashtrays, etc.

Clean up everywhere and wash all washables including your cars, carpets, furniture, and clothes. Have a fresh breath. You don't want to smell cigarette smoke anymore.

Discuss with your physician/doctor.

If you have a doctor, discuss with him about the journey so he can give you some health tips to guide you along the process.

Identifying the smoking triggers

To be successful in this journey, one of the most important things to do is to identify the things that make you smoke. It could be a group of people, feelings, activities, or situations. Understanding these factors and keeping track of their impact on you will help you a lot to overcome the barriers.

To keep track of them, you need to start keeping a journal - let's call it a Craving Journal. Use a week or more before your start date to keep track of your smoking activities. Keep record of the time, place and factors that triggered the habit.

Below are some of the things you can have in your journal to help you keep good track of the activity.

- What time did it happen?

- On a scale of 1-10, how extreme was your craving?

- What activity were you engaged in before it began?

- How was your feeling before it began?
- What did you feel after taking it?

Most of us smoke to get over some unpleasant feelings such as loneliness, depression, anxiety, stress, anger, etc. Though cigarettes help a lot to handle these feelings, we can't get over these things by destroying our health. There are healthy and effective ways we can use to manage these problems.

Doing some exercise, practising meditation, taking some healthy supplements, having a rest, sleeping, etc, can help us to manage unpleasant conditions.

The journal you keep is what will help.you to understand these situations that trigger smoking habits. Once you have taken note of them, the next thing is to figure out ways to handle these feelings without going for cigarettes. It could be by taking some energy drinks (non-alcoholic) and healthy supplements. Definitely, those feelings are inevitable. We all feel it, but it now depends on how people decide to manage the situation.

So, let's find the best healthy alternatives to get over those situations without turning to tobacco.

Dr. Sebi Diet Guide To Manage Common Triggers

Alcohol

Most people use cigarettes as a side dish when they drink. The feeling is great but we can't kill ourselves. To avoid this trigger, always avoid alcohol or places where you are tempted to take a sip. You can easily go to those places where alcohol is prohibited. Take some healthy juice and smoothies instead. Thanks to Dr. Sebi's diet. Alcohol is highly restricted. So, you will endeavor to stay on the diet.

Learn Dr. Sebi's complete guide on how to quit drinking alcohol easily in **Dr Sebi Easy Guide To Stop Drinking Alcohol**

DR. SEBI
Easy Guide To
STOP DRINKING ALCOHOL
Shobi Nolan

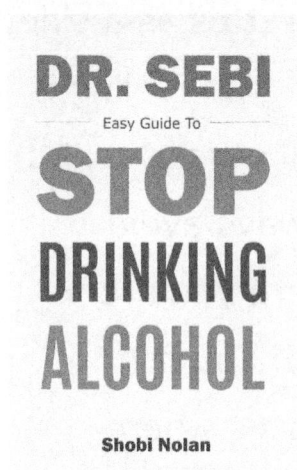

Link to kindle edition:
https://www.amazon.com/dp/B08KH2L5RZ

Avoid Smokers This Period

You know those friends or colleagues you smoke with. Tell them about your journey. Some will try to respect your decision and support you. But avoid anyone that does not accept the idea. Staying with them will lure you into the act again. Instead, learn how to practice mindfulness.

Meal Time

Many friends end their meal with tobacco. You know the meal time is ended once the light up the stick. If this is one of your habits, then you need to find an alternative. Think about taking some smoothies or fruits like apples.

Nicotine Withdrawal Symptoms

Like we state before, withdrawal symptoms are inevitable. These symptoms vary from person to person. Some can last for days, weeks, or even months. Some of these symptoms start a few hours after withdrawal.

The common symptoms are:

- Anxiety

- Restlessness
- Headaches
- Anger, irritability, or frustration
- Insomnia
- Fatigue
- Coughing
- Depression
- Constipation
- Decreased heart rate
- Tremors
- Cravings, etc

These symptoms are not easy to get over, but it can be done if we really want to do it. After all, they don't last forever. Some might stay a few days and go, while some can last up to weeks before they are completely flushed from the body.

Consequently, except some strange behaviors from you. To be on the safe side, inform your lovely ones and everyone close to you about it. That will help them to understand and tolerate any change in your usual behavior.

How To Manage Cravings

Though avoiding triggers can help to reduce the rate of cravings, you cannot completely avoid it. The interesting part is that once it starts it does not last for long. Most times, it vanishes within 10 minutes.

But how you try to handle it also determines how long it lasts. If you fix your mind on it, it will last longer than expected. So, find something to do in order to distract yourself. Also remember why you must quit smoking. Leave that environment and take a walk. There could be a trigger there.

Other things that can help you manage or avoid cravings are;

- Brushing your teeth
- Drinking a lot of water.

- Doing yoga or having little moments of meditation.

Instead of relying on nicotine replacement therapy, you can go natural by following Dr. Sebi diet. This is the healthiest means of quitting smoking.

Dr. Sebi Guide To Manage Nicotine Withdrawal Symptoms

- If you feel weak and tired, take Dr. Sebi's Energy Booster Tea
- If you feel anxiety, anger, irritability, frustration, etc, take Dr. Sebi's Nerve / Stress Relief

Herbal Tea. It helps in relaxation and relieves the nerves from stress.

- If you feel constipation, stomach pain, etc, you can take Dr. Sebi's Stomach Relief Herbal Tea

- If you have persistent cough, take Dr. Sebi's Cold / Cough Herbal Tea to relieve it.

- For decreased heart rate, you can take Dr. Sebi's Blood Pressure Balance Herbal Tea.

- For cravings, find Dr. Sebi approved fruits or vegetables to take.

All these supplements are highly effective and can help you manage all the symptoms associated with nicotine withdrawal.

Following Dr. Sebi diet and mucus cleanse can help you flush the toxins that are responsible for the symptoms faster. Thus, instead of the symptoms lasting for months or weeks, you can reduce them to a few days.

CHAPTER 5

MUCUS CLEANSE

What Is Mucus?

Mucus is an aqueous secretion produced by the cells of the mucous glands. It serves as a covering for the mucous membranes. Mucus is mainly composed of water, which is the mucin secretions.

It is an important element of the epithelial lining fluid, the airway surface liquid, which is the lining of the respiratory tract. Mucus helps to protect the lungs during breathing by trapping foreign particles and infectious agents like dust, allergens, virus, bacteria, etc.

The human body always tends to produce more mucus in order to protect and prevent the airway tissues from drying out. Thus, there is a continuous production of mucus in the respiratory system.

When foreign objects get trapped by the mucus, the mucus becomes thick and changes color most of the time. This thick mucus that is usually coughed out as sputum is known as phlegm.

Mucus also plays an important role in the digestive system. The layer formed by the mucus in the small intestine and colon helps to protect the intestinal epithelial cells from bacterial infections. It also serves as a lubricant for movement of foods through the esophagus.

Interestingly, mucus is the body's natural lubricant in females which helps during sexual intercourse. It also helps to fight against infection in the reproductive system.

Mucus And Body Health

There is a continuous process of mucus production in the body, which helps to protect the body systems from infections and also provides necessary lubrication to the body.

Thus, the presence of mucus in our body is important. When mucus traps foreign and infectious bodies, it becomes phlegm. Phlegm and excess mucus in the body is not healthy. As the body produces up to a liter of mucus everyday, it is vital to get rid of it to keep the body healthy.

Accumulation of mucus in the body is the major cause of illnesses as claimed by Dr. Sebi. So, excess mucus can be a red flag for unhealthy state of the body.

Causes Of Mucus Buildup In The Body:

Just like in snails and other animals that secrete mucus, there are triggers for the production of mucus. In human beings, the major triggers are dryness and inflammation of the body. Some factors that may lead to dryness, inflammation, and other mucus secretion triggers are;

- Dry air (environment)
- Smoking
- Allergies

- Infections
- Acid reflux
- Asthma
- Low water/liquid consumption
- Medications etc.

These factors and more contribute to excess buildup of mucus in the body. The body naturally produces mucus to ensure that foreign objects (toxic and/or infectious) don't interact with the body cells. The more we have these foreign bodies, the more the body produces mucus.

When these objects get trapped by the mucus, the mucus

becomes thick and builds up as phlegm.

Moreover, our body must stay lubricated for swift movement of particles and cells in the body. Thus, dryness of the body makes the body produce more mucus, which is the liquid the body can produce naturally.

Easy Guide For Mucus Cleanse

If you are on the Dr Sebi Diet, below are simple steps you can take to clear out and prevent excess mucus and still maintain the diet recommendations.

Hydration:

Enough liquid in the body, especially warm liquid can help drain the sinuses and thin the mucus. Thus, drinking high amounts of water can help clear out mucus from the body.

Dr Sebi recommends high intake of water. Also, most fruits and vegetables recommended by Dr Sebi diet have high water content. These foods help to keep the body hydrated and prevent excess mucus production.

Moreover, some drinks like coffee and alcohol can cause dehydration in the body. Anyone on the Dr Sebi diet must stay away from alcohol. This helps to avoid dehydration.

Expectorant:

Expectorant is known to help in clearing mucus. Expectorant loosens and thins mucus, which makes it easy to cough it out of the system.

There are some herbs in the Dr Sebi diet which can serve as expectorants. The major and most used herb in the Dr Sebi approved herbs is the Red Clover.

Red Clover is a super healthy herb which aids circulation in the body. It is a natural blood purifier, and also serves as an expectorant. It is widely used by women in treating menopause related conditions like hot flashes and lumbar spine protection.

So taking red clover can help to loosen and clear mucus from the body.

Essential Oils:

Some essential oils have been proposed to be very effective in the treatment of lung disease related symptoms. People use essential oils for the treatment and prevention of chest cold and sinusitis. Some of these essential oils can be gotten from Dr Sebi approved products like eucalyptus, oregano, and thyme.

Eucalyptus has been widely used for many years to treat coughs and reduce mucus production. It helps to loosen the mucus so it can be easily coughed out. Thus, it relieves nagging coughs.

Note: This recommendations are for adults alone.

You can learn more about mucus cleanse from **Dr. Sebi Mucus Cleanse**. It is a book that has complete step-by-step instructions on how to easily detox and cleanse mucus in a 7 days by eating healthy foods, plus action plan for using expectorant, essential oils, and hydration.

Dr. Sebi Mucus Cleanse

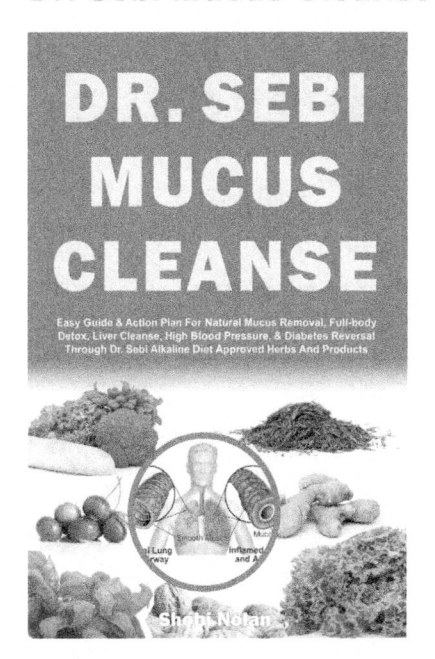

Link to kindle edition:

https://www.amazon.com/dp/B08G4Z3D8H

Link to print edition:

https://www.amazon.com/DR-SEBI-MUCUS-CLEANSE-Full-body/dp/B08GB253XW

CHAPTER 6

DR. SEBI APPROVED HERBS AND VEGETABLES

Foods with high water content and/or fiber can help the body stay hydrated, and hence prevent and cleanse excess mucus in the body. The Dr. Sebi vegetables are awesome foods with high amount of water and fiber content.

Taking these veggies will not only help you cleanse mucus, they will help your body to detox and heal naturally.

Below are some of the veggies and ways you can add them to your diet for a super healthy living.

Tomato (The Plum And Cherry)

Scientific Name: *Solanum lycopersicum*

Overview

Tomato is a popular plant grown all over the world in a temperate climate. It's widely used in different cuisines. Though it's native to western South America, China, India, the United States, and Turkey are currently the highest producers of tomatoes.

Tomato is used in many ways because of its umami flavor. It can be taken raw or cooked.

Major Compounds
Beta-carotene, lutein zeaxanthin, thiamine, niacin, vitamin B-6, vitamin C, vitamin E, vitamin K, magnesium, manganese, phosphorus, potassium

Health benefits
Heart health: Tomatoes contain high amounts of potassium and fiber. These components are important for keeping the heart healthy. Fiber helps the body to reduce cholesterol level in the blood. High consumption of potassium

helps to lower the blood pressure which is good for the heart.

Healthy bone: Phosphorus, magnesium, and vitamin C play crucial roles in the development of string and healthy bones. Tomatoes contain high amounts of phosphorus and moderate amounts of magnesium and vitamin C.

Eye health: The lutein and beta-carotene found in tomatoes are needed by our eyes to protect the retina and keep the eye free from macular degeneration.

Prevents cancer: tomatoes contain several vitamins and antioxidants such as lycopene, beta-carotene, vitamin C, etc. These components have properties that enables them to fight cancer cells and free radicals that can cause damage to the body cells.

How To Use

Tomatoes are used in many ways. It can be eaten raw or cooks. It can be used to make side dishes. Awesome for fruit and vegetable salads. Tomorrow is the major ingredient for stew. Many use it to cook soup, make sandwiches, or add it to wraps.

There are so many ways to use it. It can be used for smoothies and juice.

Nutrition fact

Per 100g

- Calories: 18 kcal
- Carbs: 3.9g
- Sugars: 2.6g
- Fiber: 1.2g
- Fat: 0.2g
- Protein: 0.9g

Side Effects

Excessive intake of tomatoes can lead to some unhealthy conditions. Some of these side effects include diarrhea, acid reflux, headache, kidney stones, lycopenodermia, joint pain, severe throat/mouth irritation, vomiting, mild spasms, dizziness, etc.

Squash

Scientific Name: *Cucurbita spp.*

Overview

Squash is a widely used food crop that originated from Mexico. Now popular in the South, North America, and Asia. India and China have been the highest producers of squash so far.

There are different types of squashes with several color variations. Squash has fed many mouths and is still feeding a lot at the moment. It is cooked and used in different dishes.

Major Compounds

Beta-carotene, lutein, zeaxanthin, thiamine, riboflavin, niacin, pantothenic acid, vitamin B6, folate, vitamin C, vitamin K, iron, magnesium, manganese, phosphorus, potassium, zinc, oleic, palmitic, and linoleic fatty acids.

Health benefits

Heart health: Fiber and potassium are important substances that help to take care of the heart. High fiber content foods help to reduce the cholesterol level in our blood. Enough intake of potassium helps the body to lower blood pressure.

Squash contains a high amount of potassium which is vital to the heart.

Cancer: squash contains important antioxidants that may help the body to prevent cancer. Some of these antioxidants reduce the growth rate of cancer cells and help to protect the body cells against free radicals.

Healthy Eye: Squash contains beta-carotene and lutein, which are important compounds for healthy eyes. They help to protect the retina and keep the eyes free from macular degeneration.

How To Use

Simply wash and peel off the skin. Then use as you desire. You can cook your squash, or roast it. Smashed and used as an ingredient for other dishes like soup.

Some squash have tough cover. To peel them off you need to put them in your oven for about 2 minutes, with the skin pierced with a fork. Or bake/cook with the skin on. Then it will be easier to remove the skin.

Nutrition fact

Per 100g

- Calories: 16 kcal
- Carbs: 3.4g
- Sugars: 2.2g
- Fiber: 1.1g
- Fat: 0.2g
- Protein: 1.2g

Side Effects

Some of the side effects associated with the use of squash include allergic reactions such as dermatitis, itching, difficulty in breathing, nasal congestion, swelling of face and lips, etc.

Onion

Scientific Name: *Allium cepa*

Overview

Onion is one of the most popular food ingredients used worldwide. Though its origin has many claims, the only fact is that onion originated from Asia.

It is widely cultivated all over the world. It can be eaten raw or cooked. Onion can be pungent to the eye when exposed. Three types of onions are predominant; the yellow onion, red onion, and white onion. All are flavorful and super healthy for use.

Major Compounds

Polyphenols, thiamine, riboflavin, niacin, pantothenic acid, vitamin B-6, folate, vitamin C, calcium, iron, magnesium, manganese, phosphorus, potassium, zinc

Health benefits

Cancer: the antioxidants in onions can help the body to fight against cancer by protecting the body cells against oxidative damage. They can reduce the growth of cancer cells, and thus, helps to reduce the risk of cancer.

Heart health: fiber in our foods helps to lower the level of cholesterol in our body. Moreover, the high amount of potassium in onions plays a vital role in the reduction of blood pressure. These properties of onions plus more ensure a healthy heart.

Osteoporosis: Calcium, potassium, and vitamin C are important to the bone. These compounds provided in good amounts by onion can help the body to develop strong and healthy bones.

Anti-inflammatory: Destroying radical cells that are toxic to the body is one of the means our body uses to prevent inflammation. The antioxidants from onions help the body to fight against these radicals.

How To Use

Onion is used to prepare most dishes.

First peel off the outer layer and wash. Dice or slice to your taste and add to your food; salads, wraps, sandwiches, soup, stew, etc. It can be taken raw or cooked. Anyway, it is super healthy for consumption.

Nutrition fact

Per 100g

- Calories: 40
- Fat: 0.1g
- Carbs: 9g
- Fiber: 1.7g
- Sugar: 4.2g
- Protein: 1.1g

Side Effects

Some of the side effects associated with the use of onions include blurred vision, dermatitis, bronchial asthma, itching, sweating, and anaphylaxis

Olive

Scientific Name: *Olea europaea*

Overview

Dominant in the Mediterranean region, olive is a very important ingredient in the Mediterranean foods. It has wonderful health benefits. Some people claim that it is the healthiest food on earth and one of the oldest known trees, thanks to its religious attachment.

Though olive is not native to the Americas, it is one of the most popular ingredients used in America, especially the oil.

Major Compounds

potassium, calcium, magnesium, vitamin E, phosphorus, sodium, polyphenol, iron, choline

Health benefits

Heart health: olive contains carbohydrates that are mostly made up of fiber. This high fiber content of olive helps the body to lower cholesterol levels.

Diabetes: research suggests that food with high fiber content strongly helps to reduce blood sugar levels.

Olive is a good source of fiber and consuming a good amount of olive will help prevent and possibly treat type 2 diabetes.

Anti-inflammatory: olive contains wonderful compounds and antioxidants that help to protect the body cells against oxidative damages, which may lead to inflammation of the body.

Cancer: the antioxidants provided by olive helps to reduce the growth of cancer cells in the body. Thus, taking olive can help one to prevent cancer cell formation.

How To Use

Olive is cultivated for different use. But most people cultivate olive for its oil which is the most used oil in the Mediterranean diet.

Nutrition fact

Per 100 g

- Calories: 146 kcal
- Carbs: 3.84g
- Sugars: 0.54g
- Fiber: 3.3g
- Fat: 15.32g
- Protein: 1.03g

Side Effects

There is no enough record on the side effects of olive. But there could be possible allergic reactions. If you have a complicated health condition, consult your physician before use.

Okra

Scientific Name: *Abelmoschus esculentus*

Overview

Okra is a widely used vegetable all over the world. Some regions call it Okro or ladies' finger. This healthy plant that originated from West Africa has a mucilaginous property. This makes most foods cooked with okra to be slimy, unless it's deslimed. One of the things mostly used to deslime okra is tomato.

This healthy vegetable is widely cultivated for food because of its nutritional values. It is used in many ways such as in making salads, soups, stews, etc.

Major Compounds
Protein, carbohydrates, fiber, vitamin K, vitamin C, thiamin, folate, magnesium, riboflavin, niacin, potassium, calcium, iron, phosphorus, zinc, flavonoids, and isoquercetin

Health benefits
Prevention of Cancer: okra contains lectin and folate. Researches suggest that these compounds strongly inhibit the growth of cancer cells. Thus, taking

enough okra can help one to prevent the risk of cancer.

Pregnancy: The folate gotten from okra helps to keep a healthy pregnancy. Lack of folate in the body may possibly lead to miscarriage.

Prevents diabetes: Test done on animals (rat) shows that okra can reduce the fat and blood sugar level in the body.

Heart health: Okra provides the body with useful fibers which can help to keep the heart-healthy. American Heart Association (AHA) suggests that food with high fiber content helps the body to reduce cholesterol level.

Osteoporosis: okra provides a high amount of calcium and vitamin K to the body. Calcium and vitamin K are very vital for the development of strong and healthy bones.

How To Use
Okra can be used in many ways. It can be taken raw, roasted, pickled, fried, boiled, or sauteed. You can

add it to your soup, salads, or other foods.

To remove the sliminess of okra in your food, try and cook it over high heat and avoid cooking in a crowded pot. You can also pickle it or cook with acidic food like tomato.

Nutrition fact

Per 100g

- Calories: 33
- Fat: 0.2g
- Carbs: 7g
- Fiber: 3.2g
- Sugar: 1.5g

- Protein: 1.9g

Side Effects

Some side effects associated with the use of okra include cramping, diarrhea, gas, and bloating.

Nopals

Scientific Name*: Opuntia spp.*

Overview

Native to Mexico, nopales is a food ingredient with important health benefits. There are about 114 species of nopales in Mexico. This highly medicinal food is not popular like other herbs such as lettuces, kale, etc, but it is common among the residents of southwest America.

It's popularly known in English as "prickly pear".

Major Compounds

Manganese, vitamin C, magnesium, calcium, antioxidants, sodium, potassium

Health benefits

Antiviral: research suggests that nopales gas antiviral properties that can be used against herpes and HIV.

Antioxidant: Nopales have a high content of antioxidants which help to protect the body cells against radical damage and reduce oxidative stress.

Blood Sugar Level: research has it that nopales have important properties that can help to regulate blood sugar levels.

Cholesterol: earlier studies suggest that nopales can lower cholesterol levels, especially LDL cholesterol.

Enlarged Prostate: Nopales may help to reduce enlarged prostate, which is a serious health condition for men. It may as well help to treat prostate cancer.

How To Use

Nopales can be eaten raw or cooked. It can be used to make juice, jams, smoothies, tea, etc.

It can be prepared with other Dr. Sebi approved foods as side dishes, salads, etc.

Nutrition fact
Per 100g

- Calories: 16
- Total Fat: 0.1g
- Fiber: 2g
- Sugar: 1.1g
- Protein: 1.4g

Side Effects

Some of the side effects associated with nopales include bloating, headache, diarrhea, nausea

Mushrooms

Scientific Name: Agaricus bisporus

Overview

With over 14,000 types, mushrooms are widely cultivated all over the world for commercial and medicinal use. China, Italy, and the United States are known to be among the highest producers of mushrooms.

The most consumed mushroom until this century remains the white mushrooms. There are many health benefits associated with mushrooms and that is one of the major reasons why it gained its popularity.

However, not all mushrooms are edible as some can be highly toxic to the body. There are over 2,000 edible mushrooms. Among the edible ones shiitake is not approved for the Dr Sebi diet. So, it's pertinent that one should avoid shitake and any other mushroom that is not edible.

Major Compounds

Protein, pantothenic acid, riboflavin, niacin, copper, calcium, selenium, potassium, fiber, vitamin D, ergothioneine, glutathione

Health benefits

Cancer Prevention: The antioxidants in mushrooms can help to prevent cancer cells from reproducing. Thus, mushrooms help the body to lower the risk of cancer.

Neurodegenerative Disease (Alzheimer's): Ergothioneine and glutathione which are majorly produced by mushrooms are claimed to be potentially useful for the treatment of Alzheimer's and Parkinson's diseases

Heart Health: Mushrooms are one of the major producers of potassium.

High intake of potassium helps to reduce blood pressure.

Diabetes: The fiber content of mushrooms can help to fight against diabetes. Fiber is known to be useful in managing type 2 diabetes.

How To Use

First trim the end of the stalk, clean, and wash before use. It can be sliced, diced, or used the whole. Though it can be taken raw, cooked mushrooms are most preferred.

Mushrooms can be used to make salads, side dishes, pizza,

scrambles, quiche, omelette, sandwiches, wraps, etc.

Nutrition fact

Per 100g

- Calories: 22
- Fat: 0.3g
- Total Carbs: 3.3g
- Fiber: 1g
- Sugar: 2g
- Protein: 3.1g

Side Effects

Dryness of the mouth or throat, rashes, diarrhea, itchiness, stomach upset, cramps, headache, nausea, vomiting, and diarrhea

Dandelion

Scientific Name: *Taraxacum officinale*

Overview

Dandelion is a herbaceous plant grown all over the world for food and medicinal purposes. It's claimed to have a myriad of medicinal properties that can be used in the prevention and potential cure for physical ailments.

Native to North America and Eurasia, dandelion is widely consumed as a nutritious food. All parts of the plant are edible, including the flower, leaves, roots, and stems.

The flowers are known to contain high amounts of phytochemicals, with the leaves rich in lutein, while the root has a lot of probiotic fibers.

Major Compounds

Vitamin A, folate, vitamin K, vitamin C, calcium, potassium, iron, manganese, polyphenols, inulin, lutein, beta-carotene

Health benefits

Good Source of Antioxidants: dandelion provides the body with a good amount of antioxidants such as beta-carotene and polyphenols which help to protect the body cells against radical damages.

Regulation of Cholesterol Levels: researches done on animals suggests that dandelion is very effective in reducing cholesterol levels. It also lowers the amount of fat in the liver, which means that dandelion can be used for the treatment of fatty liver disease.

Blood Sugar Regulation: the antihyperglycemic, anti-inflammatory and antioxidative properties found in dandelion can be useful for the treatment of type 2 diabetes.

Anti-inflammatory: chemical extracts from dandelion are claimed to be potent in the reduction of body inflammation.

Blood Pressure Regulation: potassium is known to be an effective supplement for lowering blood pressure.

Weight Loss: the chlorogenic acid found in dandelion can be effective in reducing weight and lipid accumulation.

Prevention of Cancer: Research suggests that dandelion can be highly effective in the prevention of cancer as it has the potential to inhibit the growth of cancer cells.

Immune System Boost: The antibacterial and antiviral properties of dandelion can be useful for the immune system. Research suggests that dandelion can inhibit the growth of hepatitis B.

How To Use

Dandelion can be used in many ways. Depending on how you want it, it's mostly preferred when blanched to remove some bitterness. It can be taken raw (both fresh and dried), added to smoothies, teas, and juice, or used to make salads. It can be added to soup. The root can be roasted and used as coffee.

Nutrition fact
Per 100g

- Calories: 45
- Total Fat: 0.7g
- Total Carbs: 9.2g
- Fiber: 3.5g
- Sugar: 0.7g
- Protein: 2.7g

Side Effects

There is no enough record on the side effect on the use of dandelions. But dandelion can cause allergic reactions, diarrhea, or heartburn.

Lettuce

Scientific Name*: Lactuca sativa*

Overview

Lettuce which originated from Egypt and mostly produced in China is widely known for its wonderful health benefits. Some people call it the perfect weight-loss food.

It can be used in diverse ways for various purposes, especially for medicinal purposes. In many regions, it is used for the treatment of typhoid, body pain, smallpox, rheumatism, coughs, and nervousness - even insanity, though there is no scientific backup for this claim.

There are different types of lettuce which include leaf lettuce, romaine lettuce, iceberg, summercrip, butterhead, red leaf, oilseed, and celtuce.

Note: Iceberg is not approved by Dr. Sebi.

Major Compounds

Vitamin K, vitamin A (beta-carotene, lutein, zeaxanthin), folate, iron, thiamine, riboflavin, pantothenic acid, vitamin c, vitamin e, calcium, magnesium, manganese, phosphorus, potassium, sodium, zinc

Health benefits

Prevents Dehydration: lettuce, especially red lettuce is made up of 96% water. This can help to keep the body hydrated.

Antioxidant: lettuce contains a lot of antioxidants such as beta-carotene which helps to protect the body cells against radical damage. Antioxidants play vital roles in the wholesome wellness of our bodies.

Heart Health: the presence of potassium in lettuce may help to lower the level of blood pressure.

Eye Health: The beta-carotene and other antioxidants got from lettuce help to protect the eye from macular degeneration.

Prevents Diabetes: Lettuce has a low glycemic index and zero glycemic loads which are good for those trying to lower their blood sugar, especially for managing type 2 diabetes.

How To Use

First wash the lettuce, pound on a chopping board to make it soft. Separate the leaves and dry. Then tear into smaller parts and dress.

Lettuce can be used to make smoothies, salads, and sandwiches. It can also be added to soups and wraps.

Nutrition fact

Per 100g

- Calories: 15
- Fat: 0.2g
- Carbs: 2.9g

- Fiber: 1.3g
- Sugar: 0.8g
- Protein: 1.4g

Side Effects

Some of the potential side effects associated with lettuce consumption include sweating, itching, fast heartbeat, nausea, vomiting, pupil dilation, diarrhea, dizziness, ringing in the ears, vision rashes, vision changes, sedation, and breathing difficulty.

Izote

Scientific Name: *Yucca gigantea*

Overview

Commonly known as yucca, izote is a garden plant that is native to Central America and Mexico. It is claimed to have varieties of medicinal properties. It is one of the most popular sources of saponin, a natural detergent.

Generally, it is cultivated as a houseplant, ornamental garden, herb, or food. Thus, it is used in diverse ways, especially in the treatment of illness like arthritis.

Though it can survive in different soils and conditions, it thrives most in hot semi-arid or warm climates.

Health benefits

Arthritis: According to research, the chemical extracts from izotes can potentially help in the treatment of arthritis.

Heart Health: steroidal saponins from izote helps the body to lower cholesterol level in the blood. This helps to keep the heart healthy.

Prevention of Cancer: the phenols gotten from izote can help to prevent the growth of cancer cells, and thus, eliminating any potential risk of cancer.

Anti-inflammatory: izote contains phenols like resveratrol and yuccaols A, B, C, D and E, which are known to be anti-inflammatory.

How To Use
First remove the ovaries and anthers. Then blanch for about 5 minutes. You can cook your izote

with onion, tomatoes, and chile. Bool and eat with lemon juice, or use it with egg-battered patties.

Side Effects

Some possible side effects associated with izote are upset stomach, bitter taste, vomiting, nausea.

Kale

Scientific Name: *Brassica oleracea*

Overview

Kale is one of the most popular veggies in the world. It is highly nutritious and heavily used for its medicinal properties.

It's claimed to originate from Asia Minor and Eastern Mediterranean where it was cultivated for food. Kale is best cultivated in the winter times for maximum yield.

Major Compounds

Protein, fiber, vitamins A, C, and K, folate, alpha-linolenic acid, lutein and zeaxanthin, phosphorus, potassium, calcium, zinc, carotenoids, phenols

Health benefits

Diabetes: The fiber content of kale can play an important role in the prevention and treatment of diabetes since fiber helps to regulate blood sugar level.

Antioxidants: kale contains a high amount of antioxidants which help to protect the body cells against oxidative damage.

Heart health: high intake of potassium and reduction in the consumption of sodium helps to lower the risk of high blood pressure. Moreover, fiber in our diet helps to lower cholesterol level. These properties help to take care of the heart.

Prevention Cancer: The presence of antioxidants in our body helps to protect our cells and hinder the development of cancer cells.

Healthy Eye: the lutein and zeaxanthin gotten from kale help to protect our eyes against macular degeneration. Vitamins, zinc, and beta-carotene help to protect the retina and keep the eyes healthy.

Healthy Bone: Calcium and vitamin K are very important for the development of healthy bones. Even, phosphorus and vitamin D also support the health of our bones.

Healthy skin and Hair: the human skin needs beta-carotene and vitamin A for development and maintenance of body tissues. Also, the vitamin C provided by kale helps to build and support the protein, collagen, responsible for skin and hair growth

How To Use

You can use kale in many ways. Kale can be eaten raw, steamed, or sauteed. Gently scrunch the kale leaf to make it soft. Then add it to your salads, sandwiches, and smoothies, wraps. Blend with other veggies and fruits to make smoothies and juice. Saute with onion for a side dish. You can spice it up and bake for 15-30 minutes to make your kale chips.

Nutrition fact
Per 100g

- Calories: 49
- Fat: 0.9g
- Total Carbs: 9g
- Protein: 4.3g

Side Effects
If you are battling with hypothyroidism, kale is not the best vegetable for you. Consult your physician for your diets. Excessive

intake of kale can inhibit the production of thyroid hormone.

Garbanzo Beans

Scientific Name: *Cicer arietinum*

Overview

Garbanzo beans is a nutrient-dense legume which is highly cultivated almost in all parts of the world. It is highly rich in fiber, protein, folate, iron, etc.

There are two types of garbanzo, the big size with light color, which ich predominant in the Americas and the small size with dark color that is mainly found in the Middle East and India

However, American garbanzo beans are far sweeter than the

Indian garbanzo beans. This is one of those foods that takes time to cook, but it always comes out with great taste.

Major Compounds
Protein, folate, fiber, iron, phosphorus, fatty acids, sitosterol,

Health benefits
Diabetes: Beans are known to be slow in digestion. Garbanzo beans have a very low glycerin index (GI) and glycemic load (GL). These properties help to reduce blood sugar and insulin levels. Thus, it can

be used to control the sugar level of patients with type 2 diabetes.

Heart Disease: the plant sterol in garbanzo beans known as sitosterol helps to lower the cholesterol level in the blood.

Obesity: the high fiber content of garbanzo beans can help to promote weight loss. High fiber content in a diet makes one have the feeling of fullness, and this satiating effect helps in weight loss.

How To Use

First sort the beans to remove stones and debris. Then soak overnight and cook for about 1 or 2 hours, depending on the heat you are using. Check for recipes and get directions. You can use the cooked garbanzo beans in many ways.

It can be added to your stew, soup, or salad. You can make hummus with it by blending it with olive oil, lemon juice, garlic, and tahini. Mashed and used in place of flour.

Roast and grind to make coffee.

Nutrition fact

Per 100g

- Calories: 378 kcal
- Carbs: 62.95g
- Sugars: 10.7g
- Fiber: 12.2g
- Fats: 6.04g
- Protein: 20.47g

Side Effects

Some of the side effects recorded on the use of garbanzo beans include stomach cramp, gas pains, and discomfort. The allergies associated include redness, rashes, inflammation, diarrhea, and hives.

Cucumber

Scientific Name: *Cucumis sativus*

Overview

Cucumber is a creeping vine plant that is cultivated all over the world. According to history, cucumbers originated form India before spreading to other parts of the world.

It contains about 95% water which makes it one of the best fruits/vegetables to manage dehydration. It is cultivated for both food and medicinal purposes as it contains healthy substances that are highly beneficial to the body.

Major Compounds

Calcium, potassium, magnesium, phosphorus, iron, sodium, vitamin C, beta-carotene, folate,
lutein zeaxanthin, nantothenic acid, cucurbitacin, vitamin K, vitamin B-6, thiamine, riboflavin, niacin

Health benefits

Hydration: hydration is one of the major benefits of cucumber as it is made up of 95% water. This water is super healthy as it has important electrolytes which helps to prevent constipation and maintain healthy intestine.

Healthy Bone: vitamin and calcium are very important for the bone. Calcium keeps the bone strong and healthy while vitamin K facilitate the absorption of calcium. Also, vitamin D supports the heath if the bone.

Cancer Prevention: Cucurbitacin is a nutrient know to inhibit cancer cells from reproducing and hence prevents the development of cancer cells.

Heart Health: The fiber content of cucumber helps to regulate cholesterol levels and prevent possible heart disease.

Diabetes Prevention: Cucumber has low glycerin index, which means it has low potential of increasing blood sugar. Also, according to American Heart Association (AHA), fiber helps to prevent type 2 diabetes.

How To Use

Cucumber is usually eaten raw. You can add it to your salads or sandwiches. Use it to make side dishes and have a good meal time.

For your smoothies and juice, you can blend cucumber and add it.

There is no specific limitation to the use of cucumber. You can add it to any food you feel like enjoying with cucumber. The most important thing is for it to add value to your health and also give you a great taste.

Nutrition Facts

Per 100g

- Calories: 65 kJ (16 kcal)
- Carbs: 3.63g
- Sugars: 1.67
- Dietary fiber: 0.5 g

- Fat: 0.11 g
- Protein: 0.65 g

Side Effects

Excessive amount of vitamin K may affect blood clotting. So it's advisable to consume reasonable amount of cucumber since it contains a lot vitamin K.

Some allergies associated with the consumption of cucumber include swelling and hives. Some people also report of difficult breathing. So, watch out for thethese signs.

Chayote

Scientific Name: *Sechium edule*

Overview

Chayote originated from Mexico and many parts of Latin America. Now it's grown all over the world. It's also known as choko or mirliton. It is mainly used when cooked.

Almost all part of this pear-shaped plant is edible, including the root, leaves, stem, and seeds. It contains loads of nutrients that can help transform and keep the body healthy.

Major Compounds

Potassium, vitamin C, magnesium, folate, manganese, vitamin K, vitamin B-6, zinc, quercetin, myricetin, morin, kaempferol

Health benefits

Promotes Heart Health: according to researchers, some chayote compounds help to reduce blood pressure and improve blood flow.

Also, Myricetin which is provided by the body helps to reduce the level of cholesterol in the body. Moreover, taking fiber-rich foods helps to lower the risk of heart disease - chayote is one of the fiber-rich foods.

Blood Sugar Control: the fiber content of chayote helps to promote insulin sensitivity and regulation of blood sugar.

Support Healthy Pregnancy: The folate provided by chayote helps to lower the risk of miscarriage during pregnancy.

Anticancer: the myricetin in chayote has a strong anticancer property which helps to fight against cancer.

Anti-Aging: Chayote is loaded with a high amount of antioxidants which help to protect the body cells against oxidative damage. Also, since vitamin C is verily vital in the production of collagen, the high amount of vitamin C in chayote ensures the skin stays firm and youthful.

Prevents Liver Disease: Excessive deposits of fats in the liver leads to fatty liver disease. Test tube and animal studies suggest that chayote extract can help to protect the liver by preventing the accumulation of fats in the liver.

Support Digestion: The fiber and flavonoids from chayote keep the digestive tract healthy as they keep the digestive enzymes in the gut healthy and remove wastes from the digestive tract, respectively.

How To Use

Chayote is mainly used when cooked, roasted, steamed, or fried. You can also eat it raw by adding it to your salads and smoothies.

You can add it to stews, soups, casserole dishes.

Nutrition fact

Per 100g

- Calories: 19
- Fat: 0.1g
- Cholesterol: 0mg
- Sodium: 2mg
- Potassium: 125mg
- Carbs: 4.5g
- Fiber: 1.7g
- Sugar: 1.7 g
- Protein: 0.8 g

Side Effects

Allergic reactions

Bell Pepper

Scientific Name: *Capsicum annuum*

Overview

Bell peppers are 5% carbs and 94% water, with minute protein and fats.

Native to Central America, Mexico, and South America, it is cultivated in warm climate and moist soil of about 70 - 84F temperature.

It does not burn strongly like other peppers because it does not produce lipophilic chemical, capsaicin, that is responsible for the burning sensation from peppers.

Bell peppers have different colors including orange, yellow, red, and green (when unripe).

Major Compounds

Potassium, vitamins c, b-6, e, a, and k1, folate, capsanthin, violaxanthin, lutein, quercetin, luteolin,

Health benefits
Eye Health: the carotenoids, lutein and zeaxanthin, provided in large

amounts by bell peppers protect the retina from oxidative damage.

Prevention Of Anemia: Iron deficiency is the major cause of weakness and tiredness of the body which is a result of the blood not being able to carry enough oxygen.

The vitamin C provided by the bell pepper promotes the absorption of iron into the body system.

How To Use

Bell pepper can be eaten raw or cooked. You can use your bell pepper in garden salads. It can be used as toppings on your cheese steaks and pizza. You can use it for your stuffed peppers. You can dry and powder it to make paprika spice.

Nutrition fact

Per 100g

- Calories: 31
- Water: 92%
- Protein: 1g
- Carbs: 6g
- Sugar: 4.2g
- Fiber: 2.1g
- Fat: 0.3g

Side Effects

Nausea, loose stools, mild burning sensation, sneezing, stomach pain, watery eyes

Arugula

Scientific Name*: Eruca vesicaria*

Overview

Native to the Mediterraneans, arugula is a leafy green vegetable with fresh, bitter, tart, and peppery-mustard flavor. It is popularly known is some regions as garden rocket, roquette, rucola, or colewort. It is widely used as healthy ingredient for salads.

It is super nutrition and may help the body to prevent the risk of cancer, eye damage, or osteoporosis and arthritis.

Major Compounds

Potassium, calcium, phosphorus, vitamin k, vitamin b-6, vitamin c, magnesium, sodium, thiamine, riboflavin, dietary fiber, fat, protein, vitamin a, beta-carotene, lutein zeaxanthin, niacin, vitamin e, iron,

Health Benefits

Healthy Bone: Calcium, vitamin K, magnesium, and phosphorus supplied by arugula are the major minerals for the development of strong and healthy bone. These minerals helps the body to prevent any risk of osteoporosis and arthritis.

Heart Health: Arugula contains wonderful minerals to take care of the body naturally. Arugula contains high amount of potassium, vitamins and antioxidants, with moderate amount of fiber which help to protect the heart. The fiber helps the body to lower and regulate the level of cholesterol in the blood, while the potassium reduces blood pressure.

Cancer: The vitamins and antioxidants from arugula help the body to prevent the formation of cancer cells. They also protect the body cells against radical damage. This also aids anti-inflammation.

Eye Health: The high content of vitamin A, lutein and b-carotene in arugula protect and help the eyes to fight against macular degeneration.

How To Use
First rinse with cold water and dry. In addition to the leaves and seeds, it is good to know that the young seed pods, and flowers of arugula are also edible. They can be used to make salads. It can be added to soups, or used to make sauce.

Some people also use it for their pizza.

Side Effects

Some possible side effects with excessive consumption of arugula include abdominal cramping, flatulence, and discomfort.

Turnip Greens

Scientific Name: *Brassica rapa var. rapa*

Overview

Turnip greens are root vegetables widely cultivated worldwide as food crop. It thrives better in the temperate climates. Turnip green is known as one of the best sources of vitamins and regarded as one of the healthiest vegetables in the world.

During winter and late autumn, turnip is the most common side dish in southeastern region of United States. It's fully packed with antioxidants, potassium, calcium, and fiber.

Major Compounds
potassium, phosphorus, magnesium, vitamin K, folate, vitamin C, zinc, iron, sodium, Lutein, beta-Carotene,

Health Benefits

Heart Health: Turnip contains wonderful substances to take care of the body naturally. Turnip contains high amount of potassium, fiber, vitamins and antioxidants which help to protect the heart. The fiber helps the body to lower and regulate the level of cholesterol in the blood, while the potassium is a good mineral used by the body to reduce blood pressure.

Hair and Skin Care: Vitamin C in one of the major vitamins supplied by turnip to the body. Vitamin C helps the body to build and maintain collagen. Vitamin A is vital for all body tissues including those for skin and hair. While iron helps to stop hair loss.

Healthy Bone: Calcium, vitamin K, vitamin D, magnesium, and phosphorus supplied by turnip are the major minerals for the development of strong and healthy bone. These minerals helps the body to prevent any risk of osteoporosis.

Pregnancy Care: The vitamins and minerals produced by turnip are vital to keep a healthy pregnancy. Folate in the body protects pregnant women from the risk of miscarriage.

Cancer: The vitamins and antioxidants from turnip helps the to prevent the development of cancer cells. They also protect the body cells against free radical which could cause serious damage to body cells. This also aids anti-inflammation.

Eye Health: The high content of lutein and b-carotene protects and helps fight against macular degeneration.

Diabetes: Fiber is known to help in managing type 2 diabetes as it helps to regulate blood sugar.

How To Use

First rinse with cold water, and slice as desired. Turnip can be eaten raw or cooked. You can add turnip to your salad or smoothie. It can be sauteed or boiled, and added to soups, casserole, or other dishes. Side dish for rice and beans,

Side Effects

Though turnip is a wonderful source of healthy minerals, too much consumption of it may not be healthy for the body since it contains high amount of these minerals already.

Some of the possible side effects that could be associated with the consumption of turnip include runny nose, cough, watery eyes, lip swelling and redness, sore eyes, sinus, breathing problems, etc.

Watercress

Scientific Name: *Nasturtium officinale*

Overview

Watercress is a rapid growing flowering plant that is widely used in Europe and Asia. It is native to these two continents, but has found its wide use in other regions like the Americas. It is known to be one of the oldest vegetables on earth.

It is an aquatic plant and thus, perfect for hydroponic cultivation. It is used in different delicacies and it is highly nutritious. It can be eaten raw or cooked.

Major Compounds

potassium, calcium, vitamin K, phosphorus, folate, magnesium, vitamin C, vitamin A, beta-Carotene, lutein zeaxanthin, vitamin E, riboflavin, vitamin B-6, manganese, thiamine, pantothenic acid, iron, sodium

Health Benefits

Heart Health: Watercress contains high amount of potassium, vitamins and antioxidants which may help to keep a healthy heart. High amount of potassium helps the body to reduce blood pressure.

Skin Care: Vitamin C helps the body to build and maintain collagen while vitamin A is vital for tissue development including those for skin.

Healthy Bone: Calcium, vitamin K, vitamin C, and phosphorus from watercress are essential minerals in the formation of strong and healthy bone. These minerals keeps the bones free from osteoporosis and arthritis.

Cancer: The vitamins and antioxidants from turnip helps to prevent the build up of cancer cells. They also protect the body cells against oxidative damage to body cells.

Eye Health: The amount of lutein and b-carotene in watercress is very high and they can help to protect the eye from macular degeneration.

Other Possible Health Benefits

Some people use watercress as a short-term solution for inflammation of the lungs, baldness, and sexual arousal.

How To Use
Mostly used to make salads, watercress can be used in other foods like soup, omelet, scrambled egg, pasta sauce. It can be added to sandwiches, wraps, smoothies, and juice.

Side Effects
There is no enough record on the possible side effects of watercress. It is advisable to use moderate amount of watercress, and then

watch out for any possible side effects.

Purslane

Scientific Name: *Portulaca oleracea*

Overview

Purslane is a leafy green vegetable with sour and salty taste. Wide known as weed because of its ability to survive in harsh conditions, unlike other green veggies. It is more common as edible vegetable in the Middle East, Europe, and Asia. Even the Mexicans are used to it.

It can be eaten raw as salad or used in several delicacies. Its mucilaginous property makes it perfect for soups and stews.

Major Compounds

potassium, calcium, magnesium, phosphorus, folate, vitamin B-6, vitamin E, vitamin C, vitamin A, iron, manganese, thiamine, niacin, riboflavin, zinc

Health Benefits

Anti-inflammatory: The vitamins gotten from purslane have anti-inflammatory and antioxidant properties. These properties help to protect body cells against free radicals and thus, keep the body free from inflammation. It may also be essential for cancer prevention.

Heart Health: Purslane is one of the best sources of potassium among leafy greens. Thus, may be essential for the heart, since potassium helps to reduce blood pressure.

Skin Care: Vitamin C and E the major vitamins supplied by purslane to the body. Vitamin C is known to be vital for collagen while vitamin E plays a vital role in cell regeneration. These vitamins help to keep the skin free from blemishes.

Healthy Bone: Calcium, magnesium and phosphorus provided by purslane are essential minerals for strong and healthy bones. These minerals help to to prevent and treat osteoporosis and arthritis.

How To Use

Purslane's leaves, stems, and flower buds are very much edible and they are highly nutritious. Purslane can be used in salads and soups. It is good for stir-fries. It is good to know that the fresh young leaves are the best for use.

Some people apply fresh purslane leaf on the skin to treat burns, and other skin ailments.

Side Effects

Enough data have not been recorded on the side effects associated with the use purslane.

Amaranth Greens

Scientific Name: *Amaranthus dubious*

Overview

Amaranth Greens are herbaceous edible leafy vegetables that are native to Mexico and Central America. In the pre-Columbian time, it is one of the healthiest staple foods cultivated by the Aztecs and Incas.

Nowadays, it's mostly cultivated in the tropical climate of Asia, Latin America, and Africa where it flowers from some to fall.

In the subtropical environment, it can flower throughout the year.

In India, China, and Africa amaranth is usually cultivated as leafy-vegetable. The Europeans and Americans cultivate amaranth for their grains.

Health Benefits

- The stems and leaves contain a healthy amount of insoluble and soluble dietary fiber. This is why it is highly recommended by dieticians for a weight loss program and control of cholesterol levels in the body.

- Amaranth leaves are known to contain no zero cholesterol and a good amount of healthy fats. The greens contain approximately 23 calories/100g.

- Amaranth greens are vital for complete wellness of the body as they contain adequate amounts of antioxidants, vitamins, phytonutrients, and minerals required by the body.

- Iron is one of the essential components for the production of red blood cells. During cellular metabolism, iron serves as a co-factor for cytochrome oxidase (oxidation-reduction enzyme). A fresh Amaranth green of about 100g carries 29% DRI of iron.

- Amaranth greens contain a high amount of potassium, even more than spinach. Potassium is a very important mineral in the cells and body fluids. It helps to regulate blood pressure and heart rate.

- It also contains high amounts of magnesium, calcium, manganese, zinc, and copper, which are vital components for the body cells.

- Like other greens, amaranth helps the body in preventing weakness of the bone, which is known as iron-deficiency anemia (osteoporosis).

How To Use
For the grain:

- Add to water twice the volume of the grain or 2.4 times the weight of the grain and boil.

For the leave:

- Separate the leaf and stem.
- Wash the leaf with cold water and gently pat dry with a tissue.
- Then chop before you use it in any recipe. It can also be used without chopping.

- Do not overcook the amaranth leaf so you don't destroy most of its nutrients, especially the vitamins and antioxidants.

- It can be used in soups, stews, curries, and mixed vegetable dishes.

- You can also use it raw to make juice or salad.

Avocado

Scientific Name: *Persea American*

Overview

Avocado, a fruit classified as a member of Lauraceae (a flowering plant family) is claimed to originate from south-central Mexico. It's a popular plant that is cultivated throughout the world in the Mediterranean and tropical climates.

Well known as butter fruit because of its creamy texture, avocado is a nutrient-dense fruit with a high amount of healthy monounsaturated fatty acids. It contains about 20 vitamins and minerals.

Health benefits

Nutrient-Dense: Avocado is a wonderful source of vitamins B-6, K, C, and E, folate, potassium, lutein, omega-3 fatty acid, riboflavin, pathogenic acid, niacin, magnesium, and beta-carotene.

Heart Health: a healthy cholesterol level is vital for the health of our heart. Beta-sitosterol plays a vital role in maintaining the cholesterol level that is healthy for the heart. Consuming plant sterols regularly helps a lot and avocado contain about 25mg/ounce of beta-sitosterol.

Eye Health: Lutein and zeaxanthin provided by avocado serve as antioxidant protectors in the eyes to reduce damage.

Osteoporosis: Vitamin K is very vital for the bone. Vitamin K helps to reduce the loss of calcium through urinary excretion and also facilitates calcium absorption. Taking half if avocado prices us with about 25% of the daily recommendation.

Cancer: although the true mechanism on how it works is yet to be known, researchers believe that the DNA and RNA are protected against undesirable mutations by folate during cell division. This folate helps to protect against cervical, stomach, colon, and pancreatic cancer.

Pregnancy: Folate also helps during pregnancy to reduce the risk of miscarriage and possible defects if the neural tube.

Depression: homocysteine impairs the delivery of nutrients to the brain. This substance also interferes with the production of dopamine, norepinephrine, and serotonin that controls sleep, appetite, and mood. Folate helps to prevent this homocysteine from building up.

Digestion: half of avocado contains 6-7 grams of fiber. Taking this with natural fiber helps to maintain the digestive tract and lower any risk of colon cancer.

Other health benefits of avocado include detoxification, antimicrobial action, protection and treatment of chronic disease and osteoporosis.

How To Use

It's important to know that we only use avocados in our meals when it ripens. How do you know when it's ripped? Gently press the skin. If it's soft and budge, then it's ripped. If not, give it some days to ripe.

You can use your avocados in your salads and sandwich, as guacamole and dip. The avocado oil is used for cooking and also for moisturizing the skin.

CHAPTER 7

DR SEBI FOOD LIST

Vegetables

- Arame
- Wild Arugula
- Bell Pepper
- Zucchini
- Chayote
- Wakame
- Dulse
- Nopales
- Cucumber
- Garbanzo Beans
- Hijiki
- Sea Vegetables
- Avocado
- Dandelion Greens
- Izote flower and leaf
- Kale
- Cherry and Plum Tomato
- Mushrooms except Shitake
- Lettuce except iceberg

- ✓ Olives
- ✓ Nori
- ✓ Onions
- ✓ Purslane Verdolaga
- ✓ Squash
- ✓ Tomatillo
- ✓ Turnip Greens
- ✓ Amaranth
- ✓ Watercress
- ✓ Okra

Fruits

- ✓ Tamarind
- ✓ Prickly Pear
- ✓ Peaches
- ✓ Bananas
- ✓ Figs
- ✓ Prunes
- ✓ Cherries
- ✓ Berries
- ✓ Rasins
- ✓ Currants
- ✓ Pears
- ✓ Dates
- ✓ Orange

- ✓ Grapes
- ✓ Limes
- ✓ Mango
- ✓ Plums
- ✓ Apples
- ✓ Soft Jelly Coconuts
- ✓ Melons
- ✓ Cantaloupe
- ✓ Papayas
- ✓ Soursoups

Spices and Seasonings

- ✓ Sage
- ✓ Achiote
- ✓ Sweet Basil
- ✓ Basil
- ✓ Dill
- ✓ Habanero
- ✓ Cayenne
- ✓ Bay Leaf
- ✓ Onion Powder
- ✓ Oregano
- ✓ Pure Sea Salt
- ✓ Thyme

- ✓ Savory
- ✓ Cloves
- ✓ Tarragon
- ✓ Powdered Granulated Seaweed

Grains

- ✓ Fonio
- ✓ Spelt
- ✓ Kamut
- ✓ Rye
- ✓ Tef
- ✓ Amaranth
- ✓ Quinoa
- ✓ Wild Rice

Sugars and Sweeteners

- ✓ Sugar (gotten from dried dates)
- ✓ Agave Syrup gotten from cactus (100% Pure)

Herbal Teas

- ✓ Chamomile

- ✓ Red Raspberry
- ✓ Elderberry
- ✓ Fennel
- ✓ Burdock
- ✓ Ginger
- ✓ Tila

Nuts and Seeds

- ✓ Brazil Nuts
- ✓ Raw Sesame Seeds
- ✓ Hemp seeds
- ✓ Walnuts

Oils

- ✓ Avocado Oil
- ✓ Sesame Oil
- ✓ Coconut Oil
- ✓ Grapeseed Oil
- ✓ Hempseed Oil
- ✓ Olive Oil

OTHER BOOKS BY THE SAME AUTHOR

Dr. Sebi Mucus Cleanse

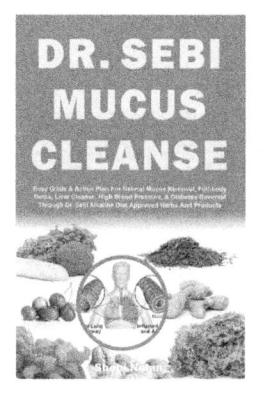

Link to kindle edition:
https://www.amazon.com/dp/B08G4Z3D8H

Link to print edition:
https://www.amazon.com/DR-SEBI-MUCUS-CLEANSE-Full-body/dp/B08GB253XW

Dr. Sebi Fasting For Weight Loss, Treatment And Cure

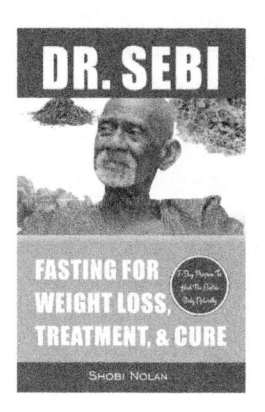

Link to kindle edition:
https://www.amazon.com/dp/B08H1HXCSN

Link to print edition:
https://www.amazon.com/SEBI-FASTING-WEIGHT-LOSS-TREATMENT/dp/B08GVGCDC2

Dr. Sebi Alkaline Diet Detox Guide For Women

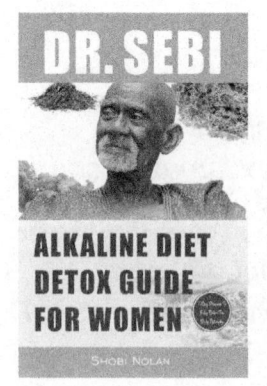

Link to kindle edition: https://www.amazon.com/dp/B08H2FSSJ5

Link to print edition: https://www.amazon.com/SEBI-ALKALINE-DETOX-GUIDE-WOMEN/dp/B08GVGD18H

Dr. Sebi Natural Blood Pressure Control

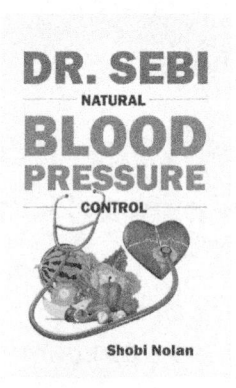

Link to kindle edition: https://www.amazon.com/dp/B08JCKFNNL

Link to print edition: https://www.amazon.com/SEBI-NATURAL-BLOOD-PRESSURE-CONTROL/dp/B08JB1XH13

Dr. Sebi Approved 3-Day Mucus Buster Diet For Women

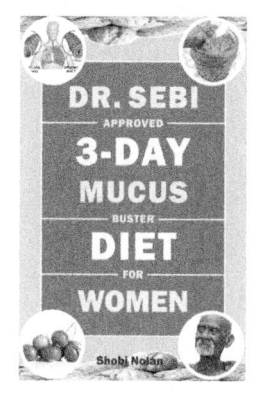

Link to kindle edition: https://www.amazon.com/dp/B08GMBD8DX

Link to print edition: https://www.amazon.com/APPROVED-3-DAY-MUCUS-BUSTER-WOMEN/dp/B08GVJTRNY

Dr Sebi 7-Day Cure For Herpes

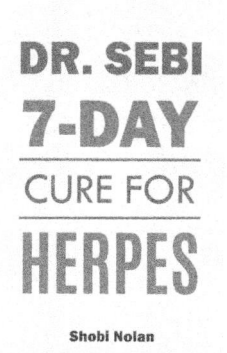

Link to kindle edition: https://www.amazon.com/dp/B08KGYVP8M

Dr Sebi Easy Guide To Stop Drinking Alcohol

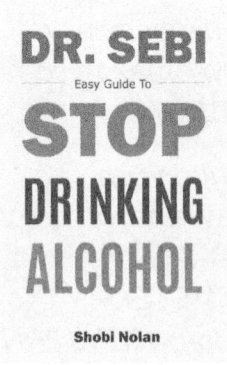

Link to kindle edition: https://www.amazon.com/dp/B08KH2L5RZ

Dr Sebi Low Cholesterol Diet

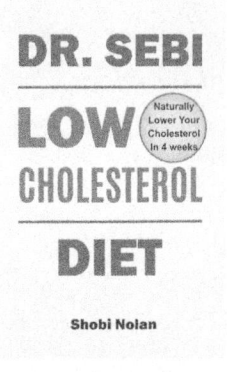

Link to kindle edition: https://www.amazon.com/dp/B08KGZZKBP

Dr Sebi Easy Way To Stop Smoking

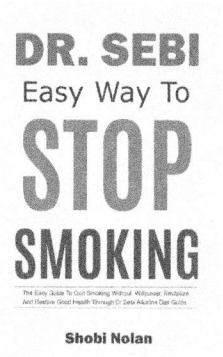

Link to kindle edition: https://www.amazon.com/dp/B08J9QNZBR

Link to print edition: https://www.amazon.com/SEBI-EASY-WAY-STOP-SMOKING/dp/B08JF5CZBZ

Dr. Sebi Diet Guide To Stop Acid Reflux

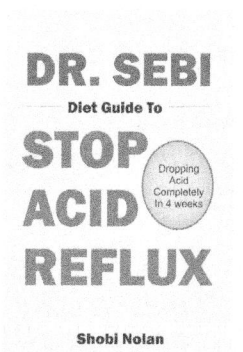

Link to kindle edition: https://www.amazon.com/dp/B08JB29WD8

Link to print edition: https://www.amazon.com/SEBI-DIET-GUIDE-STOP-REFLUX/dp/B08JF29RHF

The New Breath - Dr. Sebi's Natural Science To Stop Asthma

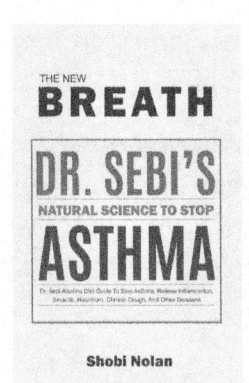

Link to kindle edition: https://www.amazon.com/dp/B08JB565XR

Link to print edition: https://www.amazon.com/NEW-BREATH-Inflammation-Sinusitis-Heartburn/dp/B08JF5CS15

Dr. Sebi Alkaline Herbal Cure In 28 days

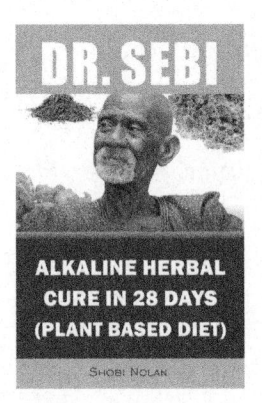

Link to kindle edition: https://www.amazon.com/dp/B08H1G3CQQ

Link to print edition: https://www.amazon.com/Sebi-Alkaline-Herbal-PLANT-BASED/dp/B08GVLWJVJ

The Dr. Sebi Diabetes Cure Book

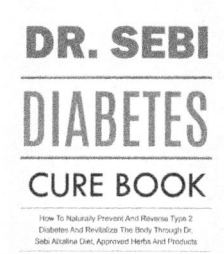

DR. SEBI

DIABETES CURE BOOK

How To Naturally Prevent And Reverse Type 2 Diabetes And Revitalize The Body Through Dr. Sebi Alkaline Diet, Approved Herbs And Products

Shobi Nolan

Printed in Great Britain
by Amazon